I0428190

The Complete Fibromyalgia Guide for Beginners

How to Conquer Fibromyalgia & Live Chronic Pain Free for Life with Fibromyalgia Diet Recipes

JACK CARTER

Table of Contents

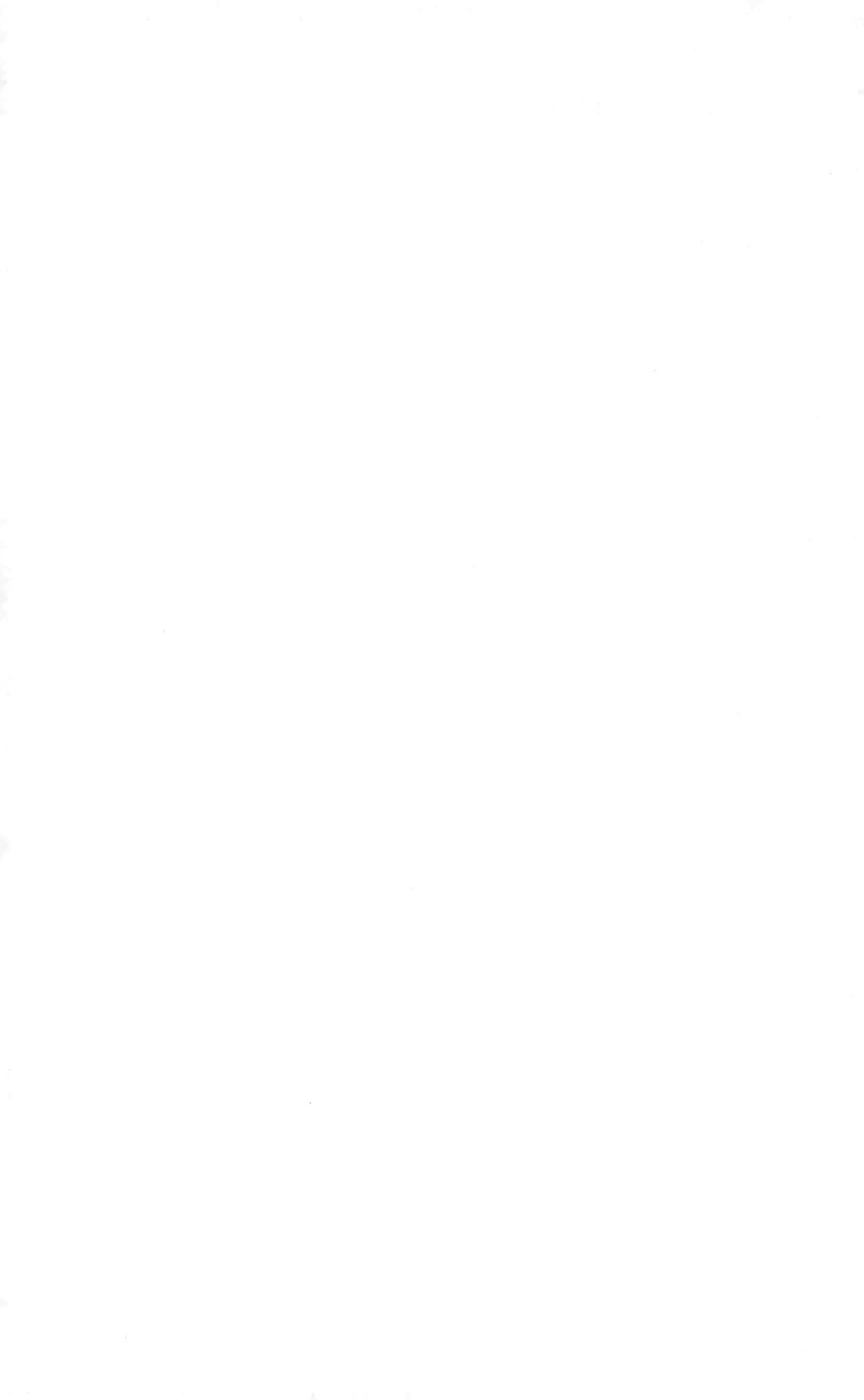

Introduction

I want to thank you and congratulate you for purchasing this book.

This book contains proven steps and strategies on how to get rid of fibromyalgia and the pain it makes you go through with delicious recipes.

It will also tell you what fibromyalgia is and its causes, symptoms, diagnosis, conventional treatments and alternative treatments. With such information, you will be able to treat the symptoms of this condition and stay away from fibromyalgia for the rest of your life.

Thanks again for purchasing this book, I hope you enjoy it! Please take some time to stop by and LIKE our Facebook page:

https://www.facebook.com/joypublishing

With gratitude,

JACK CARTER

Chapter 1

What is Fibromyalgia?

Aside from osteoarthritis, another usual musculoskeletal disorder is fibromyalgia. Not everyone understands this condition and it is usually misdiagnosed. Because of the pain and exhaustion it brings, it can make a sufferer feel isolated and depressed.

Above twelve million people in the U.S. suffer from fibromyalgia and they consist mostly of females from 25 years old to 60 years old. Compared to men, women are ten times more prone to this disease. There are some studies that reveal this is because the serotonin present in the female body is seven times lower than men. Serotonin is a neurotransmitter which overturns pain receptors.

Fibromyalgia is said to have different causes. They include genetics, stress and hormonal imbalances. Many researchers say this condition also comes from a mixture of several emotional and physical triggers.

There is also a theory by some experts saying fibromyalgia sufferers feel so much pain because their tolerance is significantly reduced. This lowered threshold may be due to the decreased effectiveness of the natural painkillers of the body like serotonin and endorphins as well as the existence of the chemical, "substance P" which intensifies pain signals. Other medical studies say fibromyalgia can be caused by a traumatized spinal cord and brain.

One theory also says fibromyalgia is due to the body's biochemical changes and can be linked to menopause or hormonal imbalances. There are also theories that say some fibromyalgia sufferers have decreased human growth hormone levels which can result to muscle pain. These theories are said to be just speculative because there is no evidence of the real cause of fibromyalgia.

There are researchers who say that a bad physical condition and stress can lead to fibromyalgia. In addition, when the muscles are slightly damaged, this causes continuous pain and exhaustion. Such theories have not at all been proven yet as well.

There are many fibromyalgia sufferers who suffer insomnia or light sleep that does not refresh them. When a person suffers sleep disorders, the serotonin level goes down so he or she loses pain tolerance. Some researchers made a study wherein they deprived some women of sleep. They found out that these women had decreased pain tolerance which can stimulate fibromyalgia.

There are also scientists who believe fibromyalgia goes hand-in-hand with low-grade depression. Recently though, issues on mental health are not anymore linked to fibromyalgia. However, it has been proven that continuous pain can make a person depressed and anxious and these worsen the symptoms of fibromyalgia.

Fibromyalgia is a rheumatic condition and it may be the outcome of genetics passed from a woman to her daughter. There are researchers who claim the genes of a person may control the way painful stimuli is processed by the body. They have a theory that fibromyalgia sufferers have genes which make them intensely respond to stimuli that a lot of persons will not identify as painful. There are a lot of these genes that are witnessed in fibromyalgia patients.

It is theorized as well that when those having such a genetic tendency experience certain physical or emotional stressors like that of a grave health problem or an upsetting crisis, the response of their body to stress is altered. Such change may lead to the body's greater sensitivity to pain.

When you suffer from fibromyalgia, this can make your body become painful all over. You will also feel so exhausted that you will not be able to function well. There are body points which become so painful and tender to touch. Your body parts may swell and you may experience disturbed sleep. You will also feel depressed or moody.

Another symptom is feeling like your muscles have been pulled or overworked even if you did not do anything to make them feel that way. Your muscles seem to ache, burn or twitch. You may also have painful joints in your back, hips, neck and shoulders. Because of this, you will not be able to exercise well or sleep soundly.

You may also suffer different symptoms with fibromyalgia such as dry eyes, mouth and nose, painful abdomen, continuous leachates, heat or cold hypersensitivity, lack of concentration, IBS or irritable bowel syndrome, incontinence, tingly or numb fingers and feet, and stiffness.

When you have fibromyalgia, you may experience feelings and symptoms the same as that of bursitis, osteoarthritis or tendinitis. Because of this, fibromyalgia is placed in the group in disorders related to arthritis. With fibromyalgia however, the stiffness and pain you feel are all over your body. In tendinitis and bursitis, the pain is focused on a certain area.

If you think you have fibromyalgia, you will need to visit your doctor as only he can make a proper diagnosis. He shall ask you about your medical history and will tell you to undergo a physical exam. You will also undergo FM/which is a blood test that recognizes markers created by the blood cells in the immune system of fibromyalgia patients.

You will be asked to undergo certain blood tests for your doctor to discount serious medical conditions. You may undergo a CBC or complete blood count, glucose test and a thyroid test.

Hypothyroidism or a less active thyroid may lead to symptoms that are like those of fibromyalgia. These include muscles aches, depression, weakness and fatigue.

You may undergo the following lab tests if your doctor wishes to dismiss other grave conditions. These tests include:

1. ANA or antinuclear antibodies

2. ESR or erythrocyte sedimentation rate

3. RF or rheumatoid factor

4. Lyme titers

5. Tests to check your levels of calcium, vitamin D and prolactin

The ACR or American College of Rheumatology outlines symptoms that fibromyalgia patients experience. Your physician may want to check if the symptoms you have satisfy the criteria of the ACR for fibromyalgia which include persistent extensive pain at both sides of your body which does goes on for three months or more. You may feel this pain in the following parts of your body:

1. On top and beneath your waist

2. Neck

3. Middle of your back

4. Lower back

5. Chest

Aside from this pain, you will also feel tenderness at different points on your body.

Your physician shall assess the severity of other fibromyalgia symptoms you may suffer like mood and sleep disorders. It shall assist in measuring the effect of fibromyalgia syndrome on your emotional and physical condition and your overall health.

Fibromyalgia has no cure and a treatment for all its symptoms is absent. To treat fibromyalgia, there are different conventional and alternative methods which have been proven to be effective. These treatments include a proper diet, exercise, herbs, home and natural remedies and behavioral techniques.

ACR says that fibromyalgia drug therapy mainly treats the symptoms exhibited by patients. There are three medications which treat this condition that are approved by the Food and Drug Administration or FDA and they are:

1. Cymbalta

2. Lyrica

3. Savella

Cymbalta as well as *Savella* are categorized as SNRIs or serotonin & norepinephrine reuptake inhibitors. Lyrica, a treatment of nerve pain which is due to diabetes, an injured spinal cord and shingles, has been shown to lessen the pain of fibromyalgia sufferers.

The pain felt by fibromyalgia syndrome sufferers can be treated by a minimal dosage of amitriptyline, Flexiril and other tricyclic medications. Aside from these, there are also antidepressants or dual reuptake inhibitors like Effexor which has positively treated the pain of Fibromylagia. Another pain reliever for this condition is Ultram.

As mentioned, fibromyalgia sufferers experience sleep disturbances and depression aside from pain. Physicians usually prescribe Zoloft, Paxil or Prozac to the sufferers of this condition so as to relieve them of the said symptoms. A recent study has shown that Neurontin, which is an antiepileptic drug, can treat fibromyalgia.

Medications found to be successful in treating the pain of fibromyalgia are NSAIDs or non-steroidal anti-inflammatory drugs which include Cox-2 inhibitors. The disadvantages of taking opioid pain relievers are: 1) they will not be effective after using them for a long time and 2) you may become dependent on them and this can result to other problems.

For those who are not comfortable with taking drugs for fibromyalgia, they can use alternative treatments as they are safer and just as effective. Even though there is no proof of their effectiveness, many sufferers can attest to their ability to manage fibromyalgia symptoms. One such alternative treatment is a therapeutic massage which works on the body's soft tissues and muscles and helps lessen muscular pain. This treatment can remove pain caused by tense muscles, muscle spasms as well as tender points. Another treatment is myofascial release therapy that manipulates different muscles and softly realigns, lengthens, softens and stretches connective tissues for discomfort to be lessened or eradicated.

Performing light intense aerobic workouts twice or thrice per week is said to help in handling fibromyalgia according to the APS or American Pain Society. Other alternative treatments to remove pain are:

1. Acupuncture

2. Chiropractic manipulation

3. Hypnosis

4. Different kinds of body massages

Aside from these alternative remedies, you should set aside some time every day to just relax. You can perform relaxation therapies like deep breathing exercises and deep muscle relaxation to minimize stress which may generate symptoms of fibromyalgia.

You should also go to bed early and at the same time every day so that your body will be able to rest and have time to repair itself.

Diet is another way to treat fibromyalgia symptoms. The following chapter will tell you what foods to choose and to avoid when managing the symptoms of fibromyalgia.

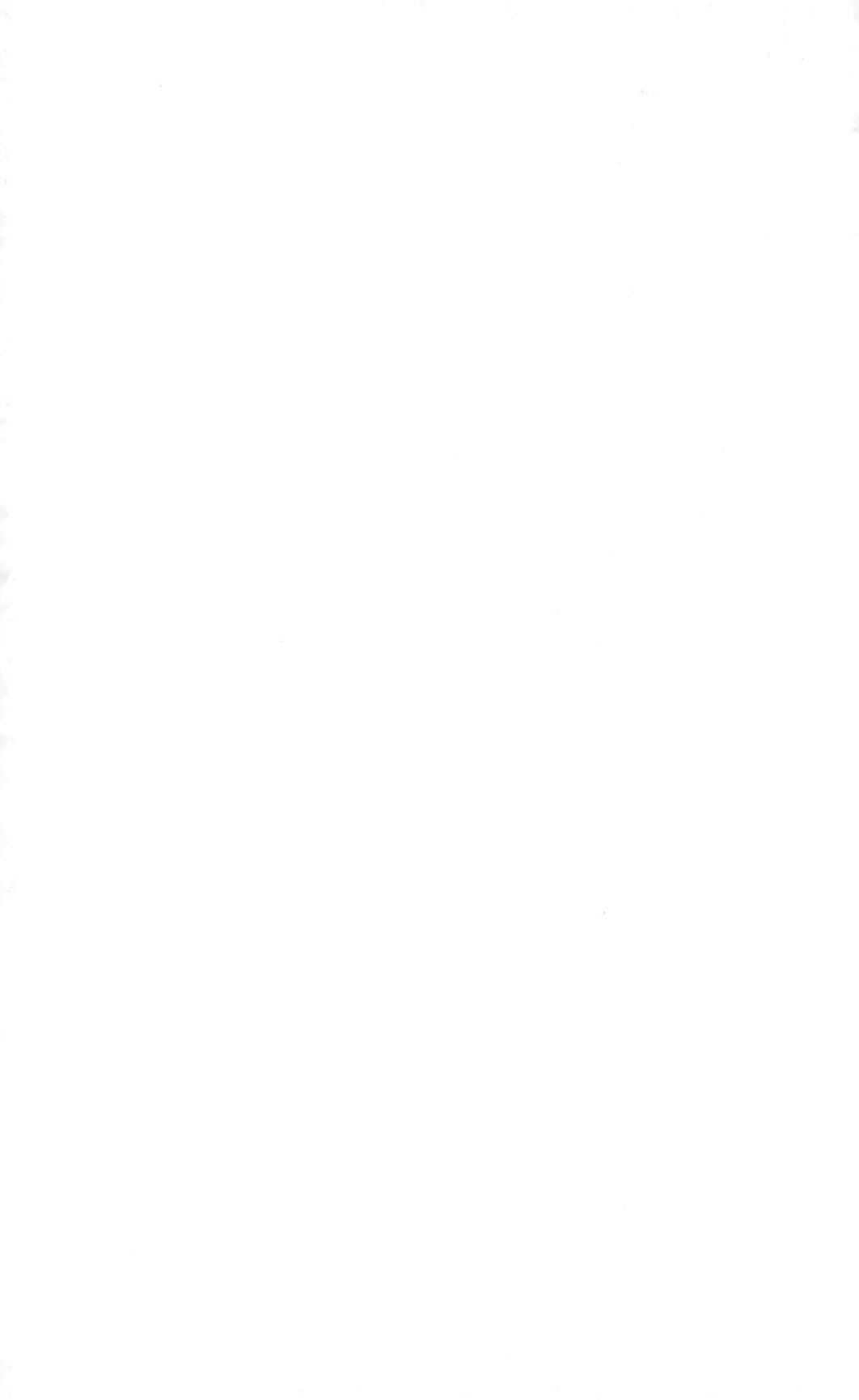

Chapter 2

Foods to Choose and Avoid When Suffering from Fibromyalgia

As mentioned in the first chapter, your fibrous connective tissues, joints and muscles become chronically inflamed when you suffer from fibromyalgia. There is no definite cause of this condition but there are theories why some people suffer it. Treating it means treating its symptoms with conventional and remedies. One of the ways to manage fibromyalgia is with food. Many sufferers become sensitive to some foods and this aggravates the symptoms. To control and eliminate these symptoms, it is vital to include certain foods in your diet.

If possible, your diet should consist of organic and fresh foods. Make sure that before you eat something, you read the labels and see that they have the words "organic" on them. Make sure they do not have additives, commercial dyes, nitrates, preservatives and trans-fat.

For the detoxification systems of your body to be less stressed, consume mostly cooked meals instead of raw foods. Cooking food will kill parasites, fungus or microbes in the body that may cause irritation.

To get enough amount of magnesium, a mineral that helps fibromyalgia sufferers, consume refried beans. You can consume the following beans as they are enriched with dietary fiber which helps get rid of toxins inside the body:

1. Black beans

2. Pinto beans

3. Kidney beans

4. Lentils

5. Chick Peas (Garbanzos)

Eat sufficient amount of fresh fruits such as grapefruit, oranges, pineapple and tangerines. Cook vegetables such as bell peppers, celery, green beans, green veggies, summer squash and winter squash.

You can consume seafood and lean meat as long as they are stir fried, baked, poached or broiled. You can consume beef, chicken, nitrate-free bacon, pork, scallops, shrimp and turkey. Eat fish that are enriched with omega-3 fatty acids such as salmon, mackerel, sardines, tuna and halibut. Cook your food with canola oil, not olive oil.

It is important to consume at least eight glasses of water every day. This removes toxins in the body and lubricates the bones, joints, tissues and muscles.

The symptoms of fibromyalgia are diverse so this means not all of the sufferers get symptomatic relief once they stay away from certain foods. It is important though to be aware of the foods to completely avoid to achieve overall relief.

Stay away from artificial sweeteners such as saccharine, NutraSweet and aspartame because they exacerbate the symptoms. Those who suffer from this condition usually possess significantly active N-methyl-D-aspartic acids (NMDA) which are pain receptors that lead to extreme pain. NMDA pain receptors present in fibromyalgia sufferers are roused by the excitotoxin aspartame. According to a study back in 2001 about pharmacotherapy, fibromyalgia sufferers who stayed away from aspartame had an overall feeling of well-being.

You should also avoid nitrates and monosodium glutamate (MSG) because these are food additives that enhance flavor as well as preserve a lot of frozen and processed foods. Nitrates serve as preservatives in bacon, bologna, ham and other cold cuts. Those who suffer from fibromyalgia have minimal tolerance levels for nitrates and MSG and these rouse NMDA pain receptors.

We mentioned including vegetables in the diet of fibromyalgia sufferers. Be aware though that there are certain vegetables of the nightshade group which cause allergic reactions, enhance discomfort and heighten pain in some sufferers of fibromyalgia. These include eggplant, potatoes, green peppers and tomatoes. These types of vegetables are nutritious so you must first determine which of them can make you experience pain or allergies. Once you determine them, remove them from your diet for a couple of months and then reintroduce them gradually one by one to see if your symptoms of fibromyalgia come back. If these vegetables do not cause allergic or painful reactions, you can continue eating them.

Fibromyalgia patients become intolerant of gluten and yeast that they can easily have gluten intolerance and yeast infections. You can find gluten and yeast in food products that are baked such as cakes, pastries and bread. When you become intolerant of yeast and you consume food with this, your body may grow fungus which can lead to muscle and joint pain.

Fibromyalgia will also make you become exhausted and this can result to digestive disorders such as gluten intolerance. "Rheumatology International" states in their April 2014 issue that intolerance or sensitivity to gluten can be the basic cause of FMS or fibromyalgia syndrome.

Aside from the foods to consume more of and avoid, it is important to stretch and workout every day, even for just 30 minutes so that your body will be strong and in good shape. Write down on your journal what you consume everyday so that you will be able to link the food you eat with the symptoms you suffer.

Chapter 3

Fibromyalgia Recipes to Try

This chapter shall present recipes you can prepare at home and include in your diet to help fight the symptoms of fibromyalgia. They contain the necessary and safe ingredients to assist you in managing this condition. Read on and enjoy.

Protein is necessary because they provide important amino acids which the body cells use to repair torn and damaged muscles and create new protein. It is necessary for the body to function properly. One of the important sources of protein is from animal meat.

Lamb Stew & Winter Crockpot

Ingredients:

- Sprig of parsley
- 1 tablespoon of butter
- 2 peeled & quartered onions
- 3 peeled & chopped garlic cloves
- 2 chopped carrots (3 inches per piece)
- 1 chopped parsnip (3 inches per piece)
- 1 chopped potato (2 inches cubes)
- 2 chopped collard green leaves (bite-sized pieces)
- 1 teaspoon of sea salt
- 1/8 teaspoon of ground black pepper
- A pinch of cardamom
- A pinch of cinnamon
- 1 tablespoon of fresh rosemary
- 2 cups of stock or water
- ½ a cup of red wine
- 8 ounces of pastured lamb stew

Procedure:

1. Place all the ingredients in a crockpot except for parsley.

2. In high setting, cook the ingredients for four to five hours. If in low setting, cook for eight to ten hours.

3. Use your fresh parsley as garnish.

As mentioned in the last chapter, you need to consume fish enriched with omega-3 fatty-acids when suffering from fibromyalgia. One kind of fish is halibut.

Roasted Halibut

Ingredients:

- 2 scrubbed and halved russet potatoes (halved lengthwise, half-inch spears
- 2 tablespoons of olive oil (extra-virgin)
- 2 quartered and seeded red bell pepper (8 half-inch wedges)
- 1 peeled white onion (8 half-inch wedges)
- ½ a teaspoon of salt
- Fresh ground pepper
- 2 tablespoons of chopped flat-leaf parsley
- 2 teaspoons of chopped lemon zest
- 1 teaspoon of dried oregano
- 1 clove crushed garlic
- 1 skinned halibut fish fillet weighing one and a half pounds and divided into four portions
- Lemon wedges

Preparation:

1. Heat your oven to 400°F.

2. Get a baking sheet that is large-rimmed and place potatoes in it.

3. Sprinkle with oil, making sure to coat the potatoes evenly.

4. Place onion and bell pepper.

5. Sprinkle with one-fourth teaspoon salt and pepper.

6. For half an hour or till the potatoes turn brown and tender, roast your vegetables. Turn potatoes a couple of times and move onion and pepper around for even browning.

7. Chop parsley, oregano, garlic and lemon zest together to create gremolata.

8. Season the fish with one-fourth teaspoon salt and pepper and two teaspoons of gremolata.

9. Take the pan from your oven and increase temperature to 450°.

10. Place the veggies to the sides.

11. Put the fish in the middle of the pan.

12. Place some of the peppers and onions on the fish and position the potatoes on the edges.

13. Roast till you see the veggies become tender and brown and the fish is smoky and then wait for another 10 to 15 minutes.

14. Sprinkle the rest of the gremolata above the halibut.

15. Place the fish on a platter along with the veggies.

16. Place the lemon wedges on top.

Instead of drinking unhealthy beverages such as colas, sodas, alcohol and caffeine, it is best to drink juices and smoothies from fresh fruits and vegetables. These have vital nutrients and enzymes to be healthy, energetic and stronger.

Raw Power Shake

Ingredients:

- 1 to 2 pieces of carrots
- 1/3 small beet
- Asparagus
- 1 to 2 cups sour fruits (berries and plums)
- 1 to 2 peeled Kiwi
- 1-inch ginger
- 1 oz. bioactive liquid minerals
- 1 bunch of parsley minus the stalks
- Cilantro
- 2 teaspoons of turmeric
- ¼ teaspoon of cinnamon
- 1 teaspoon of sea salt
- 2 teaspoons of bee pollen
- 2 teaspoons of lecithin granules
- 2 and a half cups of distilled water
- High-powered or regular blender

Preparation:

1. Place all the ingredients in your blender.

2. Pulse your blender a number of times.

3. Blend all the ingredients for a couple of minutes.

4. Serve.

Fibromyalgia sufferers can also consume a vegetarian diet because they have protein from plants and minimal saturated fats.

Such a diet has many fibrous fruits and veggies which are delicious, healthy and satisfying.

Bone-Building Minestrone

Ingredients:

- 1 tablespoon of butter
- 1 tablespoon of olive oil
- 1 clean and chopped leek
- 4 peeled and diced garlic cloves
- 5 cups of stock from chicken, beef, pork, lamb, etc.
- 2 sliced carrots (one-fourth inch rounds)
- 1 chopped red potato
- 1 diced celery stalk
- 1 red potato, chopped
- ½ a cup of diced tomatoes
- 1 ½ teaspoon of sea salt
- 1 teaspoon of dried thyme/One tablespoon of fresh thyme
- ½ a cup of kamut elbow pasta
- 1 ½ cups of cooked cannellini beans
- 2 chopped Swiss chard leaves
- 2 tablespoons of chopped parsley
- Parmigiano Reggiano

Preparation:

1. For three minutes, sauté leak in olive oil and butter in a pan.

2. Throw in garlic, potato, carrots, celery and tomatoes.

3. Add bone stalk, thyme and salt.

4. Cover the pan and allow cooking for seven minutes over medium high heat.

5. Add kidney beans, pasta and Swiss chard.

6. Allow to boil.

7. Cook for another twelve minutes over low heat with the pan covered.

8. Sprinkle your shaved Parmigiano Reggiano.

There are fibromyalgia sufferers who are sensitive to dairy products. When they consume such products, they become bloated and experience flatulence. For people who are intolerant to these types of food, they should have a diet free of dairy. This means a diet with beans, leafy greens, juice and breakfast cereals that are fortified. They should also consume fish having soft bones so as to ensure calcium intake.

Dairy-Free Fresh Baked Corn Chips with Tomato Salsa & Cucumber

Ingredients:

- 2 pieces of peeled and diced cucumbers without the seeds
- 2 big deseeded & diced tomatoes
- 1 deseeded & minced hot pepper
- 1 small peeled & minced red onion
- 1 peeled & minced garlic clove
- Lime juice
- 2 tablespoons of minced cilantro
- ¼ teaspoon of sea salt
- Olive oil
- Cut corn tortillas in triangles (bite-sized)

Preparations:

1. Preheat your oven to 375° Fahrenheit.

2. Mix all together in a clean bowl the ingredients except for the tortillas and olive oil to make a salsa.

3. Sprinkle olive oil and enough salt on the corn tortillas.

4. Bake tortillas for ten minutes or till crispy.

5. Dip your tortillas in your salsa and eat.

Fibromyalgia patients should get their share of whole grains, according to medical science. This is because whole grains are still enriched with vitamins and minerals. One whole grain is bulgur which is quick to cook. The following recipe is rich in magnesium and omega-3 fatty acids.

Mustard Greens and Bulgur

Ingredients:

- 1 cup of bulgur prepared per instructions of package directions
- 2 tablespoons of chopped walnuts
- 6 teaspoons of virgin olive oil or walnut oil (divided)
- 2 chopped shallots
- 1 teaspoon of chopped garlic
- 12 cups of mustard green (sliced thinly and without the tough stems)
- 1/3 cup of chopped pitted dates
- 3 tablespoons of water
- 4 teaspoons of white wine vinegar
- ½ a teaspoon of salt

Preparation:

1. Place your bulgur in a colander.

2. Wash bulgur with cool water.

3. Drain water.

4. Toast on medium-low heat walnuts in a dry skillet.

5. Stir walnuts till they become a bit brownish for three minutes.

6. Pour five teaspoons of oil & shallots in another skillet and cook over medium-low heat for six minutes.

7. Throw in garlic and stir for 15 seconds.

8. Throw in your dates, mustard greens and a couple of tablespoons of water and cook till the water disappears and the greens become tender. Should the pain become dry prior to the greens becoming tender, add one more tablespoon of water and cook for another four-minutes.

9. Add salt, vinegar and bulgur and cook for one minute or until heated through.

10. Pour one teaspoon of the remaining oil.

11. Sprinkle the walnuts prior to serving.

Fibromyalgia sufferers can enjoy dessert as long as they do not contain ingredients that can aggravate the symptoms of their condition. One of the desserts they can have is Crème Brule.

Crème Brule

Ingredients:

- 3 cups of heavy cream
- 2 teaspoons of vanilla extract
- 8 organic egg yolks
- ¾ cup of sugar

Preparations:

1. Heat your oven to 375° Fahrenheit.

2. Place cream in a saucepan with a heavy bottom and simmer.

3. Get a bowl, place the egg yolks and sugar in it and whisk.

4. Mix vanilla extract on the mixture.

5. Pour the hot cream slowly into the mixture.

6. For every tiny amount of hot cream added, stir the mixture for three seconds before adding the cream again.

7. Make sure the mixture does not become frothy by whisking it or else it shall not become smooth on the top when baked. Instead of whisking, stir gently as you add the yolks in the cream.

8. Get a scoop of the mixture and place in a baking dish of medium size. The mixture should form a layer that is half an inch to one inch thick. You can form the mixture into six separate oval or round ramekins, custard cups or gratin dishes.

9. Place the dish or custard dishes inside a baking dish that has high sides.

10. Put this on your oven rack.

11. Get a ladle to drizzle sufficient amount of hot water so as to arrive in the middle of the mold sides.

12. Get one sheet aluminum foil and cover the dish so that the custards shall not form a crust above.

13. For every 45 minutes, check the custards to see if they are done or not. You will feel the surface rippling if they are not yet done once you peel back the aluminum foil and wiggle the custards a bit.

14. If there are no ripples, remove the foil and wiggle all the custards.

15. If done, remove from the oven.

16. Take away the dish from the bigger dish of water.

17. Allow to cool for half an hour.

18. Refrigerate overnight prior to serving.

There are many fibromyalgia sufferers who were able to control pain and other symptoms by eating gluten-free foods. Gluten is a natural protein from barley, rye, wheat, oats, spelt and other grains. When you want to have a diet free of gluten, this means you also have less of the following:

1. Barbeque

2. Battered foods

3. Canned vegetables with sauces

4. Cheese mixtures

5. Crumbs

6. Flavored tunas

7. Frozen dinners

8. Frozen vegetables with sauces

9. Ice cream

10. Malted milk

11. Meat pies

12. Mustards

13. Pasta

14. Pastries

15. Pickles

16. Pizza

17. Salad dressings

18. Soups

19. Soy sauces

20. Starches

21. Stuffing

22. Thickeners

23. Tofu

Here is a recipe that is gluten-free and uses buckwheat which is very nourishing and energizing:

Buckwheat Cracker or Nut Bread

Ingredients:

- 2 cups of soaked & sprouted buckwheat
- 1 cup of soaked almonds
- 1 cup of sunflower seeds that are soaked in one tablespoon of olive oil
- Juice of half a piece of lemon
- 1 teaspoon of salt
- 1 teaspoon salt
- Tomato (optional)
- Red bell pepper (optional)
- Cilantro (optional)
- Carrots (optional)
- Celery (optional)
- 1 tablespoon of olive oil (optional)
- Garlic (optional)
- Spices (optional)
- Herbs (optional)

Preparation:

1. For 12 hours, soak your buckwheat.

2. For another 12 hours, rinse, drain and sprout buckwheat inside a colander.

3. For 12 hours, soak sunflower seeds and almonds and rinse and drain.

4. Put all your ingredients inside a food processor.

5. Process till you come up with a smooth preparation.

6. Place on teflex sheet and spread to ¼-inch thickness (any shape).

7. Dehydrate at 105 °.

8. After four hours, put off the sheet and place product on the mesh trays.

9. Keep on dehydrating till you get your desired dryness.

According to research, people residing in the Mediterranean undergo minimal incidence of cancer and cardiovascular disease. This is due to the kind of food the inhabitants consume which consists mainly of fruits, grains, nut, olive oil, seeds and vegetables. Rather than red meat, the people consume more of fish. The Mediterranean diet is good for fibromyalgia sufferers. Here is a Mediterranean salad dressing you can mix in your salad.

Salad Dressing Made of Green Onion

Ingredients:

- 1 cup of olive oil (extra virgin)
- ½ cup of Lakanto
- ¼ cup of apple cider vinegar
- ¼ teaspoon of sea salt
- 6 green onions

Preparation:

1. Place all your ingredients in your blender.

2. Blend till smooth and a bot thick.

Bean Salad

Ingredients:

- 1 cup of dried kidney beans which have been soaked overnight
- 3 cups of fresh water
- 2 -inches of the sea vegetable called kombu
- 1 teaspoon of sea salt
- 1 cup of fresh, trimmed green beans that have been cut into two-inch pieces
- 2 1-inch summer squash rounds
- 1 small peeled & diced red onion
- 1 pint of halved cherry tomatoes
- 5 fresh thinly-sliced basil leaves
- 2 tablespoons of apple cider or white vinegar
- 1/8 teaspoon of fresh black pepper (ground)
- 1 tablespoon of local honey
- ¼ cup of olive oil

Preparation:

1. Throw away the water where your beans have been soaked.

2. Place your fresh water and beans in a pot and boil.

3. Remove foam that rises.

4. Place your kombu and cover the pot.

5. Simmer for one hour.

6. Add your sea salt.

7. Cook for half an hour or till the beans become soft.

8. Boil water in another pot that has a steamer basket.

9. For five minutes or till tender, steam your green beans.

10. Place green beans in a bowl.

11. Do the same procedures with your summer squash.

12. Mix together all the vegetable ingredients along with your cooked beans.

13. In another preparation, combine and whisk your remaining sea salt, apple cider vinegar, pepper, olive oil and honey.

14. Combine this with your bean salad.

15. Marinate overnight in your fridge.

According to a study last 2004 which "The Townsend Letter" presented, for three months, 18 fibromyalgia patients switched to a raw vegan diet. They had reduced pain, better sleep, minimal depression and more mobility. However, when they went back to consuming cooked food, their symptoms eventually returned. Here is one raw food diet recipe you can try out.

Buckwheat with Cabbage & Corn

Ingredients:

- 1 to 2 tablespoons of unrefined and organic butter, ghee or coconut oil
- 2 cups of corn kernels
- 3 cups of chopped cabbage
- 1 large chopped onion
- ½ of red pepper that is minced
- 4 cups of water or veggie stock
- 1 ¼ teaspoon of sea salt
- ¼ teaspoon of pepper
- 1 tablespoon of Fajita seasoning
- 2 cups of roasted buckwheat
- ½ a cup of minced parsley

Preparation:

1. Except for your parsley, sauté all your veggies in your butter, ghee or oil for five minutes.

2. Add water or veggie stock, seasoning, pepper and salt.

3. Boil and then add your buckwheat.

4. Allow to simmer for twenty minutes.

5. Put off heat and put in your folded parsley.

6. Cover for ten minutes before serving.

For fibromyalgia sufferers who want to eat only soup at dinnertime to control their weight, here is one recipe that they can follow.

Black Cod & Soba Noodle Dashi

Ingredients:

- 5 cups of water
- 3 grams of Bonito flakes
- 1 strip of kombu which is 5 to 6 inches long
- 2 thinly-cut carrots (diagonal)
- 2 inches peeled & minced ginger
- 1/3 cup of tamari or shoyu that is free of wheat
- 2 tablespoons of mirin
- 3 to 4 ounces of soba noodles
- 2 to 3 thinly-sliced shitake mushrooms
- 12 ounces of black cod or sable fish that is cut into quarters
- 3 to 4 chopped bok choy leaves
- 3 minced scallions
- 1 tablespoon chopped parsley

Preparation:

1. Combine together in a four-quart soup pot bonito flakes, kombu and water.

2. Boil, cover and allot to simmer for ten minutes.

3. Take away the bonito flakes and kombu and discard water.

4. Combine carrots, mirin, ginger and shoyu.

5. Cook for three minutes.

6. Add shitake mushrooms and soba noodles.

7. Cook for a couple of minutes.

8. Add bok choy and sable pieces.

9. Cover and allow to simmer for seven minutes.

10. Place in separate bowls with a fish piece in each bowl.

11. Add parsley or scallions as garnishing.

Conclusion

Thank you again for purchasing this book!

I hope this book was able to help you to learn more about the crippling disease which is fibromyalgia. You do not have to live in constant pain and isolate yourself from the company of other people. With a little bit of knowledge and some discipline with regards to your diet, you can greatly reduce the symptoms of this debilitating disease.

The next step is to use the knowledge you gained from reading this book and start making a positive change in your life. Just because you have fibromyalgia that does not mean you have to live with it your entire life.

Finally, please remember to LIKE our Facebook page in order to find other resources and upcoming promotions:

https://www.facebook.com/joypublishing

With sincere thanks,

JACK CARTER

One More Thing...

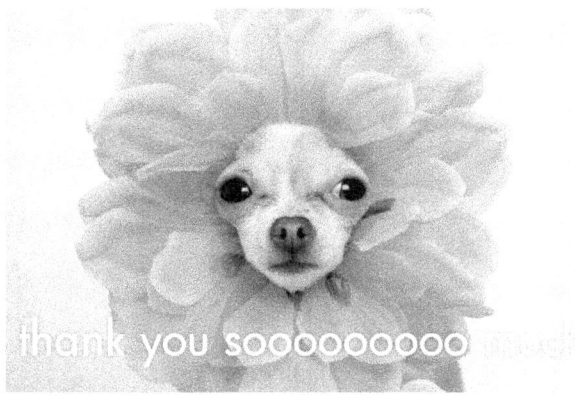

Source: Wikipedia

If you believe that this book is worth sharing, would you please take the time to let others know how it affected your life? If it turns out to make a difference in the lives of others, they will be forever grateful to you, as will I.

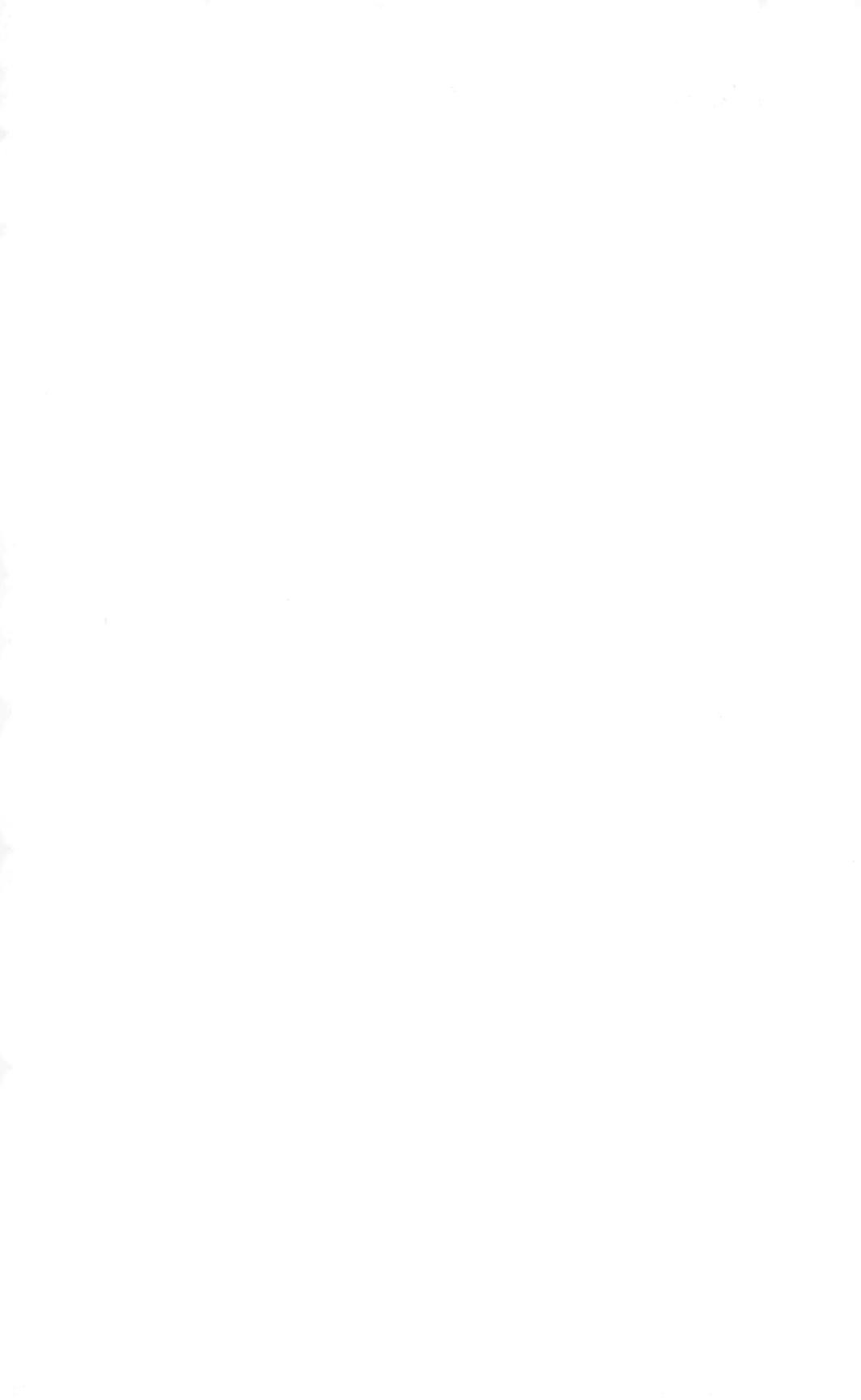

www.ingramcontent.com/pod-product-compliance
Lightning Source LLC
Chambersburg PA
CBHW070507290526
45790CB00003B/1138